THE
POWER
IN MY PULSE

**AN ATHLETES JOURNEY THROUGH
EPILEPSY, LOSS, AND RESILIENCE**

IMANI SCOTT-THOMPSON

The Power in My Pulse:
An Athletes Journey Through Epilepsy, Loss, and Resilience
By Imani Scott-Thompson

Violet Life Publishing

ISBN:
Softcover: 978-1-967081-37-0
Hardcover: 978-1-967081-36-3

DEDICATION

For my mother, Kelly Scott and godfather, Kenny Smith.
Your love, guidance, and unwavering support have carried me through times I never thought I could face. You have been my anchors, support, courage and strength.

For my younger sister, Giavonna Scott.
Thank you for being such an amazing understanding sister. You're forever by my side through it all. I appreciate you and your selflessness.

For my Neurologist, Stephen Hantus, M.D and epilepsy mentor Leigh Goldie.
You both have helped me navigate the complexities of my epilepsy and it's journey. The confidence, encouragement, and wisdom have gotten me a long way.

TABLE OF CONTENTS

THE EARLY BATTLES

My childhood was anything but ordinary. From the moment I was born, epilepsy was a constant presence, casting a shadow over my early years. While other children were carefree, I had to navigate a world where unpredictability, medicine and caution were my cohorts. The seizures, the hospital visits, and the unspoken fear that lingered in the background made my life a series of adjustments and compromises.

Living with epilepsy meant that my childhood was outlined by limitations. Simple activities that others took for granted, like sleeping on your stomach, playing outside on a hot summer day, or even playing video games were fraught with risk. I remember the frustration of sitting on the sidelines during recess, watching my friends run and play while I felt so trapped. My mom, forever attentive, worked tirelessly to ensure I could still enjoy a semblance of normalcy throughout my childhood. Despite her best efforts, the reality of my condition was always present, a constant reminder of my vulnerability.

My family was my refuge. We were a close-knit unit, bound together by love and the shared responsibility of managing my condition. I was blessed enough to have my grandmother as my registered nurse both at home and in the hospital, always there to reassure me and keep me safe. My mother, with her astounding strength, became my backbone, managing not only my needs but also the emotional toll that my epilepsy and losing my father had placed on all of us. I owe her the world for the time she has put in to make sure I was well taken care of. No matter how many hospital stays, she still remains by my side without a complaint. My younger sister Giavonna, played her part as well, learning from a young age how to be cautious and understanding of my condition. She has never judged me or complained when she had to sacrifice her time when I had a seizure. When bad seizures occurred, she was always by my side, front and center wanting to help. Together, we formed a protective loving cocoon, one that allowed us both grow and thrive despite the many challenges I faced.

While epilepsy added complexity to my life, school provided a welcome escape. Academically, I excelled, finding that the structure and predictability of the classroom suited me well. Learning came easily to me, and my grades were always above average. School became a place where I could momentarily set aside my condition and focus on something I could control. However, I often felt like an outsider, different in ways that others couldn't understand. While my classmates worried about grades and friendships, I was silently managing a condition I kept hidden from nearly everyone. It wasn't until adulthood that I began to openly share my struggle with epilepsy.

MY BODY, MY BATTLES

E pilepsy has been a part of my life since the very beginning. I was born with it, and from as early as I can remember, it has shaped the way I experience the world. The diagnosis became a defining part of who I was, influencing every aspect of my childhood and beyond. This isn't a disorder you can easily compartmentalize or disregard, it infiltrates every facet of life from the physical to the emotional, and even the spiritual. Physically, epilepsy is an exhausting condition. My body often feels drained, as if the energy that fuels others is always just out of reach for me at times.

It wasn't until adulthood, around age 20, when I found out what was actually causing my epilepsy. Polymicrogyria is an abnormal brain development of the brain before birth, in which the brain develops to many folds and are unusually small. Since this disorder is so under recognized, it can at times be hard to diagnose. Intellectual disability, motor dysfunction, and speech disturbances are a few of many symptoms that can occur in individuals with Polymicrogyria. My particular case is very rare I cannot have the preferred brain surgery, because my seizures cannot be recorded as intended. My seizures have to be recorded on an electroencephalogram but unfortunately happen when my brain chooses, not on command.

Epilepsy patients have an 161% increased risk of death compared to the general population, but yet still lacks in research, funding, and public awareness. Imagine living in fear about what can happen to you before, during, or after a seizure, I just never know. The feeling is almost impossible to explain to anyone about the physical and mental abuse that my body endure, and when people continue to ask and I cannot give answers the more frustrating it can be. A healthy brain powers at about 75-80 pulses of energy per second depending on the individual, when having a seizure that brain power rises rapidly to 500 pulses of energy per second, just take some time to think about that.

This constant fatigue is intensified by the struggle to sleep, a battle I feel I am constantly losing. Sleep, when it does come, is rarely restful. I lie awake at night, my mind racing, unable to find the peace that sleep should bring. The weight of knowing that I am caught in this constant sleepless cycle, only adds an additional level of anxiety. The medications, too, are a constant presence in my life. From a young age, I became accustomed to the daily ritual of taking multiple pills several times a day.

These medications are supposed to control the seizures, to give me some semblance of a normal life, but they come with their own set of challenges. They often leave me feeling groggy, disconnected, and even more fatigued. Yet, they are "necessary", as I am told. The act of taking these medications, of needing them to function, is a daily reminder that my body is different, that my life is governed by a condition I didn't choose.

One of the most challenging aspects of living with epilepsy is the unpredictability of seizures. They strike at random, disrupting whatever semblance of normalcy I might have been holding onto. The randomness is perhaps the most insidious part of it all the uncertainty, the not knowing when or where the next seizure will hit that creates a constant undercurrent of fear and fretfulness. Will it happen at the store? At work? In front of friends? The fear of embarrassment, of being seen in such a vulnerable state, is almost as debilitating as the seizures themselves. Although I may not know the day or time a seizure may come, I am able to identify when a seizure is going to happen soon, also known as an aura, where as other individuals with epilepsy may not. I am blessed enough to have those warning signs, so many other individuals with epilepsy who do not get auras have difficulties living average lives like driving a car for instance.

The injuries that result from these seizures can be severe. I've experienced bruises, cuts, and even broken bones over the years. Physical scars that serve as reminders of the battles my body has fought. The physical pain is often overshadowed by the emotional toll. Each seizure serves as a stark reminder that my body is not fully my own, that at any moment, it can betray me in ways I cannot prevent. The feeling of losing control, of being at the mercy of my own body, is a heavy burden to carry.

Mentally and emotionally, living with epilepsy is a relentless challenge. The lack of consistent sleep wears down on my psyche, amplifying the effects of depression that have shadowed me for much of my life. Having depression can be massive, it's a deep, pervasive sense of hopelessness that can make even the smallest tasks feel overwhelming. It's difficult to stay positive when your body and mind are at odds, each day feeling like a battle to maintain some resemblance of normality. The medications, though "necessary", are a constant reminder of my condition. Each pill is a small symbol of the limitations I must navigate, in which my life is different from those around me. There's a sense of isolation that comes with this disorder knowing that no matter how much I try to fit in, there's always this part of me that sets me apart, that makes my experience fundamentally different from others. It's a lonely feeling, one that's difficult to articulate to those who haven't lived it.

During my childhood and even my teenage years, I kept my epilepsy a closely guarded secret. My friends and family were unaware of the struggles I was facing because I didn't want to be seen as different or weak. In a world where fitting in seemed so important, I was terrified of being labeled, of being treated differently because of something I couldn't control. So, I hid it. I became adept at concealing the signs, at putting on a brave face even when I felt anything but brave.

When I felt an aura, a warning sign that a seizure was approaching, I would quietly slip away to a secluded area where I could endure the seizure alone, away from prying and judging eyes. The aura was both a blessing and a curse; it gave me enough time to find a safe place, but it also filled me with dread, knowing what was coming. The secrecy became a way of life, isolating me further and adding another layer of complexity to an already difficult condition. The fear of someone finding out, of seeing me in such a vulnerable state, was paralyzing.

Managing epilepsy during an already turbulent time in my life only heightened my struggle. It wasn't just the physical toll it took on my body, the mental and emotional weight that seemed to grow heavier with each passing day.

The seizures, the medications, the sleepless nights these are my constant companions, making an already difficult existence even harder to bear. However even in the face of all these challenges, I've learned to keep moving forward, finding strength in the resilience that living with epilepsy has demanded of me. Resilience is something I had to learn through many trials and road bumps. Each day, I've had to muster the strength to keep going, to not let epilepsy define every aspect of who I am. It's a battle, one that I fight every day, but it's also a testament to the human spirit's capacity to endure, to adapt, and to overcome adversity. Through it all, I've come to understand that while epilepsy is a part of me, it doesn't have to be all of me.

MY MISSING PIECE

As a young child there was so much I wanted to experience like riding on a rollercoaster, playing outside with my friends on a hot summer day, or even going to haunted houses. Although I couldn't experience some things as a young child, outside of having epilepsy I did still get to enjoy a blissful young life. My parents and grandparents did everything in their power to ensure I lived as close to a normal life as possible, within the limits of what they could control.

Then, at the age of 12, my world was irreversibly altered. My father, who had been one of my greatest sources of strength, was suddenly shot and killed. His death was a blow that recoiled through every aspect of my life, deepening the challenges I already faced with my epilepsy. The loss of my protector, a guide, and the person who had helped me navigate a world that was often unforgiving is a constant pain that still lingers. Him and I had just repaired our relationship, and I was stripped of so much needed time with him.

In the days that followed, the reality of his death began to set in. I remember seeing him after he was murdered, a sight that would forever be engrained into my mind. The image of my father, lifeless lying in his pool of blood, was something I could never have prepared for as a child. It was that moment that shattered my innocence and thrust me into a world of trauma and pain that I was too young to understand. The grief was suffocating, and the weight of it was unbearable. I felt as though my world had come crashing down, and with it, my sense of security and happiness.

My father had been the one who introduced me to basketball, a sport that eventually became my passion. Initially I had no interest in basketball, I was a cheerleader and was very much so happy with that decision but my father not so much. After his death, I struggled to find the motivation to keep playing, I did not pick up a ball for months. Every time I stepped onto the court, I was reminded of him, his laughter, his guidance, his annoyance, and the way he believed in me. The joy I once found in basketball was overshadowed by the pain of his absence, and the game that had once brought us closer now felt like a constant reminder of what I had suddenly lost.

As the weeks turned into months, I began to experience the effects of the trauma more acutely. The depression set in, a deep and pervasive sadness that I couldn't shake. I was just a child, trying to process the loss of my father while still dealing with the challenges of living with epilepsy. The nightmares started soon after, vivid and terrifying dreams where I relived the night of his murder over and over again. The post-traumatic stress was real, and it made every day a battle. I became withdrawn, shutting out the world as I tried to cope with the pain. Multiple suicide attempts caused me to be in psychological inpatient care. My mother did her best to support me, but losing my dad had left a void that nothing at that time could fill.

In the wake of his death, I was forced to confront the harsh realities of life head-on. The safety net that had been so carefully constructed around me was gone, and I had to learn how to cope with grief and trauma while still managing the daily battles of epilepsy. It was a time of profound struggle, but also one that would ultimately shape my resilience and determination.

The loss of my father left a gaping wound that I didn't know how to heal. At just 12 years old, I was thrown into a world of pain and confusion that I was unequipped to navigate. The grief was all-consuming, and I found myself drowning in a sea of emotions that I couldn't understand or control. In the aftermath of his death, I became a shadow of the person I once was, and the coping mechanisms I developed were more destructive than constructive.

Rage was the first emotion that took hold of me. I was angry at the world, at the man who took my father from me, lack of control, and at the unfairness of it all. That anger festered inside me, growing stronger each day, until it became a part of my very being. I lashed out, but unfortunately that anger was only directed toward my mother because she was the next closest loving person to me. I felt abandoned, lost, and completely alone in my pain. The world had shown me its darkest side at a very young age, and I had no idea how to deal with it. I internalized that rage, turning it inward in a way that was both harmful and dangerous.

She bore the brunt of my pain, my frustration, and my help-lessness. I blamed her for things that weren't her fault, and I pushed her away when she tried to help. I was angry at the world, but she was the one who was there, trying to hold me together as I was slowly falling apart piece by piece. Despite everything I was putting her through, my mother never gave up on me. She saw the pain behind my anger, and rather than responding with anger of her own, she responded with love and an unwavering amount of support. She put me through different therapies, searching tirelessly for something that could help me heal. It wasn't easy for either of us, the process took work. There were days when I resisted every attempt she made to reach me, but she never let me go. Her strength became a lifeline I didn't even realize I needed.

Through all the turmoil, our bond grew stronger. My mother's persistence, her willingness to fight for me even when I couldn't fight for myself, built a foundation of trust and love that has only deepened and carried over into adulthood. Today, we are closer than ever, our relationship forged in the fires of shared pain and the journey to healing. Her love and support has moved me in many ways. She is my confidante, my supporter, my heartbeat, and my constant source of strength; I am and will be forever grateful for mommy.

LEARNING TO STAND IN THE STORM

C utting became my way of dealing with the pain I couldn't express. It was momentous, something I could control when everything else felt so out of control. The physical pain provided a temporary release from the emotional agony that overwhelmed me day and night. I hid the scars from everyone, too ashamed and afraid to reach out for help. Each cut was a manifestation of the turmoil I felt inside, a cry for help that I didn't know how to voice. I had learned to hide my physical and emotional pain behind many barriers.

The sadness that followed was suffocating. Depression became a constant companion, wrapping itself around me like a heavy blanket that I couldn't shake off. I often found myself consumed by thoughts of suicide, convinced that the only way to escape the pain was to end it all. My attempts were desperate and terrifying, a reflection of just how lost I felt after my father was abruptly taken from me. Each time, I was pulled back from the brink, but the darkness remained, lingering in every part of my mind, waiting for another chance to drag me under. Despite the darkness, I eventually found strength in the lessons my father had taught me. His belief in me, his unwavering support, and the love he had shown me in those early years became the foundation upon which I began to try to restore my life.

In the midst of this darkness other than my mother, there were two things that kept me from completely losing myself: my godfather and basketball. After my father's death, my godfather stepped in and pulled me from the thin thread that I was barely hanging onto. He became a source of strength and stability in my world, that felt painful and uncertain. He didn't try to replace my father, no one could, but he did offer me the guidance and support of a father that I so desperately needed. His presence in my life became a lifeline, something I could hold onto when everything else seemed to be slipping away.

My godfather introduced me to basketball in a way that my father hadn't had the chance to. He took me under his wing, spending countless hours in the gym with me, teaching me the fundamentals of the game from the ground up. Those long nights in the gym became a sanctuary for me, a place where I could channel my anger, my sadness, and my pain into something positive. Basketball gave me a sense of purpose, a reason to keep going when everything else felt meaningless. It was therapy in a sense, a way to focus my mind on something other than the emotional turmoil that threatened to consume all of me.

As I practiced, I began to see the results of my hard work. My godfather pushed me, challenged me, held me accountable, and believed in me even when I didn't believe in myself. He saw the potential in me, not only as a basketball player but as a person who could rise above the circumstances life had thrown at them.

His steadfast support and the discipline of the game gave me a renewed sense of strength and determination. For the first time since my father's death, I felt like I had something to fight for, something to strive toward.

Basketball eventually became more than just a sport for me, it was my coping mechanism for my grief, and a way to channel my emotions into something constructive rather than destructive. On the court, I could forget about the pain, the loss, and the anger, and shift my focus on the game if only for a little while. The focus required to play, to improve, to win, gave me a break from the chaos going on inside my mind. Being a part of the game became my outlet, my escape, and ultimately, my recovery.

The journey wasn't easy, and I can honestly say I am still actively on that journey. Every step forward was met with setbacks, as the grief and depression diminished and flowed, sometimes overwhelming me with their intensity. There were days when even basketball couldn't lift the weight from my shoulders, when the gym felt like a lonely place, and the sound of the ball bouncing on the hardwood only echoed the emptiness I felt inside. Yet, I kept going. I kept pushing through the darkness, clinging to the moments of light that my godfather and basketball provided.

In time, I began to see that the very things that had once threatened to destroy me were also the things that were making me stronger. The rage that once consumed me became fuel for my drive on the court. The sadness that had weighed me down became a source of empathy and understanding, not just for myself but for others who were also struggling with something in their personal lives. The pain that had once seemed unbearable was slowly being transforming into resilience.

My godfather's influence was and still is immeasurable, words cannot begin to describe how grateful for him I am. He has taught me more than just how to play the game of basketball, he taught me how to compete on and off of the court, how to survive, and how to turn my pain into something powerful without sabotaging myself. Under his guidance, I learned that I could take control of my life, even when so much of it felt uncontrollable at the time. His belief in me gave me the strength to believe in myself, to see that my life had value and that I could overcome any obstacles in my path. When I didn't believe, he most certainly did.

The journey through grief and trauma was long and laborious, filled with both setbacks and triumphs. The unhealthy coping mechanisms I had once relied on as a young teenager, gradually fell away as I found healthier ways to deal with my emotions as a more mature teenager. The cutting stopped, the suicide attempts decreased, and slowly, the constant anger began to dissipate. In their place, I found a renewed sense of purpose, a determination to live my life in a way that would honor my father's legacy and the lessons my godfather and mother had instilled in me.

The process of healing wasn't linear, and there are still days when the pain feels as fresh as it had on the day my father died. Nonetheless I learned healthier coping mechanisms, to find strength in the very things that had once threatened to break me. I learned that resilience reveals itself in the painful moments that threaten to stop you, but you keep pushing forward anyways. Through it all, basketball remains my constant, a reminder that even in the darkest of times, there is always a way to find light.

Basketball wasn't my only athletic outlet. I discovered passion in other sports as well, like softball and track and field. Track became secondary sport alongside basketball, giving me a new space to release the pain inside of me. Over time I thrived in the sport , even setting school records in the 4x4 relay that still stand today. Pushing my body to the limits to cross the finish line gave me a satisfaction that words never could.

Running track also carried its own painful weight. At the start of each race my heart would pound and tears would form in my eyes, but not because of nervousness of the race. The sound of the official triggering the starter pistol before the race took me back to the moment I lost my father. That sound haunted me but I never let it hold me back. Despite the barriers I still thrived.

Athletics was a way to transform my pain into something less self-destructive. Sports helped shape me and give me the tools to grow through adversity with a level headed mind. The strength, discipline, and the will to keep moving despite when it hurt gave me the much needed mindset to maneuver through my journey.

THE STRENGTH OF STUDY AND ATHLETICS

ACADEMIC QUEST

Education has always been a cornerstone of my life, my mother was very strict when it came to academics. From a young age, I found solace in the structure and rhythm of school. It was a place where I could channel my energy and focus on something within my control. While many of my peers might have viewed school as just a routine part of growing up, for me, it was a way I could focus on something else other than my brain deformity.

From the very start of my academic journey, I was determined to excel and be at the top of my class. My grades were consistently strong, rarely every dipping below a 3.5 GPA throughout elementary, middle school, high school, and majority of college. Obtaining a certain grade point average served great importance to me, it was a testimony to my durability and determination. I was deeply committed to my education, it was a way I could have full control of something in my life. Every A on a report card was a small victory, a sign that I could be at the top of my class regardless of my disorder.

In addition to maintaining high grades, I was also inducted into national academic honor societies at a young age. These societies recognized my hard work, they were communities where I could connect with other students who shared my passion for learning. Being a part of these groups reinforced my sense of belonging in the academic world and motivated me to keep pushing myself to new heights. One of the highlights of my early academic career was winning a science fair, a moment that remains etched in my memory. Although I was always at the top of my class I was my worst critic, that victory gave me much a needed confidence boost. I had built a operational toy vehicle with mostly recyclable materials that operated by a propeller I designed, it would work by wind or electric. This project required hours of research, time, experimentation, and dedication. As I stood beside my display, explaining my work to the judges and peers, I felt a deep sense of pride. This was a moment where my hard work and intellect were recognized at a young age, and it gave me the confidence to pursue more challenging projects in the future.

My interest in engineering began early on, around age 7, and it quickly became clear that I had a natural aptitude for it. Even as a child, I was fascinated by how things worked or how I could innovate them. I would often take apart household items anything from radios to kitchen appliances not out of mischief, but out of a genuine desire to understand the mechanics of things. My mother, recognizing my curiosity, encouraged my exploration, providing me with tools and kits to safely indulge in my experiments. These early experiences laid the foundation for my future studies in engineering and sparked a lifelong passion for innovation and problem-solving.

In middle school, my academic prowess became even more apparent. Transferring middle schools from Emmanuel Christian Academy to Litchfield Middle School I was now able to take engineering courses and on the basketball team. I was also given the opportunity to take high school courses at Firestone High School, a challenge that I eagerly embraced. Walking over to the high school each day, I felt a sense of pride in being a step ahead and having early access to my then future high school.

These advanced courses set me up to be a grade ahead, a tribute to my hard work and intellectual capabilities. Although I had the option to graduate high school a year early, I made the conscious decision to stay in my grade and graduate with my class. This decision was not made lightly, but it was important to me to experience my senior year of basketball. I needed that year to develop more confidence before playing at the collegiate level. I knew I was academically ahead, but I valued the social and emotional connections I had formed with my teammates and coaches, we had become a family.

High school was a time of significant academic and personal growth for me. My participation in engineering competitions became a major focus. These competitions were intense, requiring not only a deep understanding of engineering principles but also creativity, teamwork, and accountability. I relished the challenge, spending countless hours perfecting my designs and solutions. The satisfaction of seeing my hard work pay off was immense, especially when I won some of these competitions.

Each victory was a validation of my skills and a reminder that I could excel in a field that I was deeply passionate about.

Not only was I passionate about the field, I also recognized there weren't many African-American women in the field. With noticing that, I wanted to someday help increase our representation. One of the most significant honors I received during this time was being named the best engineering student my senior year, an award that recognized the top engineering student in Akron public schools offering engineering. This award was the crowing point of years of dedication, and it was an incredible feeling to be recognized for my efforts, especially being a minority. More than just recognition, it affirmed that my hard work truly paid off and that I possessed the merit to thrive in the engineering industry with my peers.

While academics were a major focus, my love for engineering extended beyond the classroom, I was a part of engineering and robotics club. I continued to engage in personal projects, often spending my free time enhancing or learning how different objects work. The thrill of taking something apart, understanding its mechanics, and then improving it, was something that has never grown old for me. This hands-on experience was invaluable, allowing me to apply the theoretical knowledge I gained in school to real-world situations. Each project was a learning experience, teaching me not only about engineering, but also about persistence, creativity, and the importance of critical thinking. All highly valuable and usable transferable skills that can be used in the workforce.

Looking back, my academic journey was not only just a series of achievements and awards. The journey was a lifeline that provided me with structure, purpose, and a sense of identity.

In a world where so much felt uncertain, where my health was a constant source of anxiety, school was a place where I could succeed and where my efforts were rewarded. The challenges I faced in my academic pursuits were different from those posed by my epilepsy. They were challenges I had control of, I could tackle head-on, with hard work and purpose. With each success, I proved to myself and others that I was capable of great things, despite the obstacles in my path.

My academic success also laid the groundwork for the person I would become. It taught me the value of hard work, the importance of perseverance, and the rewards that come from pushing myself to be the best. These lessons extended far beyond the classroom, influencing how I approach most challenge in my life. Whether it was dealing with the unpredictability of my epilepsy or navigating the complexities of personal relationships, the discipline and focus I developed in my academic journey were always there to guide me.

Moreover, my academic achievements provided a sense of normalcy in a life that was anything but ordinary. While my health challenges set me apart in many ways, my success in school allowed me to feel like I was on equal footing with my peers. It gave me something to be proud of, something that was mine alone, and something that no one could take away from me. My academic journey was a true testament to how strong and disciplined I had to remain in order to balance both school, sports, losing my father, and epilepsy. Through all of that I still was able to obtain four degrees: an Associate of Science in Engineering, Associate of Arts in Life Sciences, Bachelor of Science in Public Health, and Master of Public Health.

As I moved forward in life, the lessons I learned during my academic journey continued to resonate. The discipline, focus, and passion that drove me to succeed in school became the same qualities that helped me navigate the challenges of sports and real life. Although the path wasn't always easy, I knew that I had the tools, mindset, and support to overcome whatever obstacles are ahead of me. My academic journey was just the beginning a foundation upon which I would build a life of persistence, passion, and perseverance.

MY GREAT ESCAPE

Basketball wasn't always the refuge it eventually became. As a child, I had a different set of interests that included soccer and cheerleading. I loved being a cheerleader, finding joy in the rhythm and camaraderie of the sport. My father, however, wasn't too keen on the idea of his daughter being a cheerleader. For years, he gently suggested that I try basketball, but I was adamant in my refusal. I didn't see myself in the game, believing it was more suited for boys, and besides, I was content with my current sports I was involved in. However, around the age of eight, my father made the decision for me. He told me I was done cheering and to give basketball a try. Initially, I didn't enjoy it I wasn't good at it, the workouts we did in the summer time were too hard, and I was only there because of him. I felt out of place, awkward, and unsure, but I persisted because I knew I didn't have much of a choice.

For three years, I played in leagues and attended a basketball summer camp annually, gradually improving but never fully embracing the sport yet. Then, when my father was suddenly killed and taken from me, I quit basketball altogether for a few months. The pain of playing a game that I had only ever played for him was too much to bear. Each time I picked up a ball, it reminded me of his absence, and the grief was too overwhelming. Knowing that he wouldn't be on the sidelines at my games anymore impacted me significantly. As the months passed, I found myself drawn back to the sport. There was a reason he had been so adamant about me playing, and I needed to find out what he seen in me to make him feel that way.

Around this time is when my godfather stepped into my life consistently, he seen the difficulty I was having with losing my father. He quickly began to treat me as his own daughter, teaching me the game of basketball, coping mechanisms, and many other life lessons. With his constant leadership, basketball evolved from a painful reminder of loss into a powerful outlet for my grief. The pain of not seeing my father in the bleachers during games still stands, but my god father gave me the proper tools to translate that pain into my game or academics. Basketball slowly became everything, I could transform those negative emotions into something less destructive.

The long nights in the gym full of blood, sweat, and tears with my godfather were absolutely life-changing. He pushed me in ways I didn't know I needed, helping me release the negative energy that had been swallowing me whole. While my peers were out partying and indulging in the typical teenage distractions, I was in the gym, honing my skills, and focusing on finding myself again every single day.

My godfather's influence helped me see basketball not just as a game, but as a way for different avenues. I knew I wanted to play collegiate basketball, and I understood the level of dedication and effort it would take to get there. In middle school,

I became a starter, and that first taste of success was a turning point. It was an indication to the hard work I had put in, especially since I had started playing much later than many of my teammates. By the time I entered high school, basketball had become an integral part of my identity. As a freshman, I started on the freshman team, junior varsity, and dressed varsity, dominating both the freshman and JV levels. My sophomore year saw me starting on JV, but after just five games, where I averaged 30 points in just two and a half quarters, my coach had seen enough and informed me that JV was too easy. I wouldn't get any better by dominating everyone so he removed me. Shockingly, I was upset with that decision because I knew that would come with very limited playing time on varsity, as our team was full of great players with much experience.

Junior year was when I finally became a full-time varsity starter, though I struggled a lot with confidence. I was still grappling with the weight of my father's death, and the pressure I placed on myself was immense. Trying to deal with those emotions had caused me to be extremely hard on myself, afraid to shoot the ball when my team needed it the most, as one of the best shooters on the team I was scared of missing. A bad quality I had to grow to learn to get over if I ever wanted to succeed in the sport at a high level.

By my senior year, everything started to come together. I led North East Ohio in points and steals, a remarkable achievement that earned me spots in two all-star games, multiple awards, and the satisfaction of helping my team win our fourth conference championship in a row. Although my coach and I bumped heads often he is one of the most influential people in my life. Basketball was more than just a sport for me, it was and still is a major part of me, a way to honor my father's memory, and a source of immense pride. Each accomplishment on the court was a reminder of how far I had come, not only as a player, but as a person who had endured unimaginable loss and found a way to turn that pain into some type of purpose on and off of the court.

THE PURSUIT OF EXCELLENCE

Playing basketball most certainly taught me a great deal of discipline, not just in terms of physical fitness or skill development, but in life as an entirety. From the moment I picked up a basketball, I was introduced to a world where discipline was a requirement and a necessity. Whether it was the early morning practices, the grueling conditioning sessions, or the relentless drills, basketball demanded that I show up. Success required being mentally prepared to push beyond my limits, to endure when my body and mind were screaming for rest. The discipline I developed on the court became a foundation upon which I built much of my life.

Teamwork was one of the first lessons I learned in basketball, and with it came an understanding of how discipline is integral to working effectively with others. Basketball is a sport that thrives on the collective efforts of the team. Individual talent can only take you so far; it's the disciplined coordination, the shared understanding, and the mutual trust among each teammate that leads to success. I quickly realized that my actions on the court affected not only my performance, but the entire team's outcome especially as a leader. This awareness required me to be disciplined in my approach to practice, games, and even how I conducted myself off the court. When playing a sport it is not just about you, it is about how each individuals discipline contributes to the larger goal of the team.

Time management was another critical aspect of the discipline I gained from sports. Balancing practices, games, and training sessions with schoolwork and other responsibilities required a level of organization that was both challenging and essential. I had to learn how to prioritize, how to make the most of every hour in the day, and how to ensure that neither my academic pursuits nor my athletic commitments suffered. This was not an easy task, but the structure of my daily routine helped me develop a disciplined approach to managing my time, one that has continued to serve me well in all aspects of my life.

Academics, too, played a significant role in shaping my discipline. The nature of academic work, with its deadlines, long-term projects, and rigorous standards, required a different kind of discipline. In school, I couldn't afford to procrastinate or let my focus waver; the consequences of missing a deadline or failing to prepare adequately for an exam were too significant. Each assignment, each exam, was a challenge that required careful planning and disciplined execution. Through my academic journey, I learned the importance of diligence and toughness.

There were times when the material was difficult or when balancing school with basketball and epilepsy felt overwhelming, but I had to keep pushing forward to achieve my long term goal. The discipline I had developed on the court translated into my studies, I approached each academic challenge with the same determination and focus that I brought to basketball. This crossover between sports and academics created a synergy that enhanced my abilities in both arenas.

Working through academic challenges also taught me the value of disciplined problem-solving. Whether it was a complex math problem or a research project, I learned to break down the tasks into manageable steps, to approach each one methodically, and to keep pushing forward until I reached a solution. This disciplined approach to problem-solving became a key tool in my education and in how I approach life currently. My god father also taught me how to split my goals up into quarters, as an athlete if you translate life issues to in-game issues it makes things much easier to digest.

Perhaps the most profound way that discipline has shaped my life is in the management of my epilepsy. Living with epilepsy requires a level of discipline that extends beyond academics and sports it saturates every aspect of my daily life. The unpredictability of seizures means that I have to be constantly vigilant, strategically managing my activities to avoid potential triggers. This has required a deep, ongoing commitment to self-discipline, something that I've had to cultivate over many years.

The discipline I've developed through basketball, academics, and managing my epilepsy has become a cornerstone of who I am. It has shaped my approach to challenges, both big and small, and has given me the tools to persevere through adversity. Discipline has taught me that success isn't always about talent or intelligence, showing up every day, putting in the work, and staying committed to your goals, no matter the obstacles in your path are the stepping stones. This sense of discipline has also instilled in me a deep sense of accountability to myself, to my friends, to my family, and to my future.

I know that my actions have consequences, and that the choices I make today will shape the person I become tomorrow. Whether it's on a court, on the track, in the classroom, in my career, or in my daily life, discipline has been the guiding force that has helped me navigate the complexities of my journey. As I move forward, I carry this discipline with me, knowing that it is the foundation upon which I can build my dreams. It is the discipline that will continue to push me towards excellence, to strive for more, and to never settle for anything less than my best self.

Managing epilepsy has been an ongoing challenge, especially when it comes to sleep and medication. Despite my efforts, epilepsy often disrupts my sleep, leaving me with only about four to five hours of rest each night. I've participated in epilepsy sleep studies to better understand this, but the struggle unfortunately persists. Medication is another area where I've faced significant challenges. Taking a significant amount of pills a day can be overwhelming, and I dislike the way they make me feel. Staying disciplined with my treatment is a work in progress, and it's something I continue to navigate daily.

The sheer volume of pills fourteen a day to be exact can be daunting, and I've often struggled with the side effects they bring. The medications can make me feel lethargic, disconnected, and not quite myself, leading to a deep-seated frustration and the inability to do normal life task on a day to day. There are times when I simply cannot bring myself to take them as prescribed, feeling overwhelmed by the constant reminder of my condition. Despite knowing the importance of adhering to my medication regimen, the physical and emotional toll it takes has at times lead me to stop taking them altogether. It's a daily battle, one where discipline is key, but even with the best intentions, it remains a work in progress. The process of finding the right balance between managing my health and maintaining a sense of normalcy is ongoing, and each day presents new challenges.

FACING ADVERSITY IN COLLEGE AND EARLY ADULTHOOD

THE COLLEGE
EXPERIENCE

Moving to college was a significant turning point in my life. Leaving behind the familiar surroundings of home and stepping into the unknown world of college was both exciting and overwhelming. Attending Dakota College wasn't my initial choice. I was verbally committed to Butler University, but at the end of junior year they had gotten a coaching change. I had numerous academic and basketball scholarship offers from universities of all levels, and the process of deciding on a school after Butler became overwhelming due to the sheer number of options and only having so many visits. Once August came around I told myself I would take the next school to offer me, it happened to be Dakota College at Bottineau. North Dakota brought an extreme culture shock, going from a city to a small town was difficult for me to wrap my head around. The environment was completely unfamiliar; the temperatures were below zero, and there was not much around. Despite the cons I feel fortunate to have had the opportunity to learn many new things like the Native American culture and experience how people live beyond the city. This change provided an opportunity for growth, learning how to be more independent since I was so far away from my family and how to adapt to change quickly.

Though I was there on a basketball scholarship, I wanted to make the most of my opportunity, especially since my education was fully paid for. I decided to double major in both Engineering and Public Health, aiming to maximize the benefits of being a full scholarship athlete. Looking back, I realized how fortunate I was to have such a rare opportunity, and I was determined not to waste it. Many people would assume that managing academics, athletics, epilepsy, a job , work study and a social life would be overwhelming, but for me, it was the perfect challenge. At Dakota College, I embraced every part of my life. I genuinely loved everything I was doing, from studying to playing basketball. The Bottineau community was and still is incredibly supportive. My coaches, teammates, and professors all seemed invested in my success, and this made all the difference in my growth. Having that kind of support system helped me develop valuable relationships. With so much on my plate, it was crucial to learn how to prioritize and organize my life efficiently.

I then moved on to Valparaiso for my last two years. Even though my time at Valpo was far from perfect, it taught me many lessons that reached beyond the court or track. Playing at that level you quickly realize how much mental toughness is truly required of yourself. Every day was a test whether it was in practice, the classroom, or navigating situations that pushed me outside of my comfort zone. Those experiences forced me to grow, learn how to adapt when things didn't go as planned, and to hold myself accountable in moments where it would've been too easy to fold.

On the floor, I was often asked to step up in the biggest games, whether that meant being the leading scorer when the team needed offense, or locking down the player on defense. Playing on ESPN and seeing my name pop up on the app were surreal experiences, things I had always dreamed of as a child. Living out my dreams reminded me that through the struggles, I was living out moments many never gotten the change to.

At the same time, I built memories and relationships that I will always value. Some of my closest friendships came from my time there, and even though I didn't always enjoy the day to day, I can look back and appreciate what I have gained from it. Valpo gave me a perspective that no other stop in my journey could've offered, it showed me both the hard side of chasing a dream and the fulfillment that still comes with pushing through it

THE FRUITS OF MY
EFFORT

My first two years of college were remarkable in wats I could never have imagined. As a freshman, I lead my team to my school's first ever trip to the national tournament. That milestone went beyond a simple win for the program, it signaled that we could compete against anyone team. Walking into the national tournament for the very first time, knowing our team had made history, filled me with a sense of pride I still carry with me today. With relentless effort, sacrifice, and dedication, barriers were broken and history was made.

Becoming only the third women's basketball All-American in Dakota College history stands as another unforgettable highlight of my career. An honor that I never took for granted, reflected upon my performance and the hard work of my coaches and teammates who pushed me daily. Each shot, each game, each practice represented thousands of hours of preparation. Representing my school at the highest level of competition left a chip on my shoulder, it gave me the mindset that no one in the nation could guard me.

My accomplishments didn't stop there though. I became known for my outstanding three point shooting, not just at my school, not just in the conference, but across the entire nation. I broke and set the single season three point record with 143 makes, an achievement spanning across NJCAA Divisions I, II, and III. Holding the number one national rankings for three pointers made, and the number three national ranking for points per game kept me motivated. When I became the first women's basketball player out of the entire NJCAA to hit 12 three pointers in a season, the moments started to become surreal. That night I was unguardable scoring 45 points, and more importantly, that game alone gave me the confidence boost that I needed.

More recognition followed my efforts. I was named NJCAA National Player of the Week, becoming the first women's basketball players in my schools history to earn this distinction. That honor marked a new chapter for the program, and I took great pride in setting that standard. In addition, I earned Mondak conference player of the week three times, recognition that highlighted my consistency. Selection of first and second team all-region honors acknowledged the impact I had against teams we faced, while being chosen for the All-Academic Team twice proved that I could balance many things and still be successful.

Scoring over 1,000 points marked another groundbreaking milestone during my time there. I was yet again, the first women's basketball player there to achieve this record. These accomplishment carried special meaning because it went far beyond numbers, it represented my legacy I left behind.

After two years at Dakota College, it was time to move on. I transferred to Valparaiso University, excited about the new challenges and opportunities that awaited me. However, my time at Valparaiso turned out to be much more difficult than I had anticipated. The balance between academics and athletics became more demanding, being at a private school and being a NCAA division I athlete. At Valpo, basketball required more of my time and energy, leaving less room for academics and other aspects of my life. I quickly adapted to balancing the demand of everything, but I still was far from comfortable for many other reasons.

INVISIBLE BATTLE
BEHIND THE SUCCESS

D espite my dedication, my experience at Valparaiso was far from perfect. Unfortunately, I cannot say I particularly cared for my time there. My head coach made life difficult for me, and I had to deal with her devious behavior. This was a harsh reality to face, especially only being one of three black players on the team. As an athlete, I had always been taught that hard work and dedication would be rewarded, but my efforts at Valparaiso seemed to go intentionally unnoticed by my head coach. No matter how hard I worked, or how great I played I felt I couldn't win her over. She was very manipulative and caused many other players to have a negative college experience. My assistant coaches were much more supportive, and they continuously vouched for me, recognizing the effort and skill I brought to the team. I formed close bonds with them, but despite their backing, my head coach refused to see my potential or value.

This experience wasn't limited to the basketball court. The Valparaiso community itself could also feel unwelcoming at times. Being in a predominantly white environment, I faced discrimination both in subtle and overt ways, even from professors. Coming from a middle class background and then suddenly being surrounded by so many individuals that come from wealthy families was eye opening. Being pulled over while driving on numerous occasions for no valid reason, it all slowly started to become too much. The weight of these challenges began to take its toll on me, mentally, emotionally, and physically.

The stress I experienced at Valparaiso began to affect my health in profound ways. My epilepsy, which had been relatively under control with medication at that time, started to worsen due to the constant stress I was under. The emotional strain of dealing with a toxic coach and community triggered more frequent and severe seizures. My depression deepened, I slowly was losing control of myself. I found myself in a dark place, feeling overwhelmed and physically sick. My body was breaking down, and mentally, I was at one of my lowest points. There were times when I felt like giving up completely was the easiest way out.

During this period, I questioned everything my abilities, my purpose, and my future. It was difficult to see a way out when I was constantly battling both external and internal struggles. I remember nights when I would lay awake, thinking about how far I had come, only to wonder if it was all worth it or was it a waste of time. The pressure to perform, combined with the lack of support from my coach and the isolation I felt in the community, made it unbearable at times. Nevertheless even in my darkest moments, there was something inside me that refused to quit.

In the end, what kept me going was the realization that I had a responsibility to myself. I had worked too hard to let anyone or anything take that away. Despite everything I was going through,

I couldn't let my struggles define me. I knew I had to push through and finish what I had started. With the support of some of my closest friends and teammates, I got through it.

Earning my degree became a symbol of my determination. I proved to myself that I could overcome the obstacles that were placed directly in my path. Graduating from Valparaiso was one of the most fulfilling moments of my life, I had prevailed over circumstances that were so close to defeating me. A huge weight had been lifted from my chest. I had managed to rise above the negativity, the discomfort, and the health challenges. Even though my time there was filled with hardship, I still had the opportunity to meet and experience some amazing individuals and good moments with my teammates. Although I had a rough two years there I still was able to go to Ireland and experience basketball overseas. I learned that adversity would always be a part of life, but it didn't have to dictate the outcome. I had the power to shape my future, and no one could take that away from me.

PICKING UP THE PIECES

SEEKING HELP AND
FINDING SUPPORT

My senior year was a turning point in my life, but not in the way I had hoped. Instead of the excitement of closing one chapter and stepping into the next, it became one of the most challenging and painful periods I had ever faced. As my health began to decline, both physically and mentally, I found myself at a breaking point. I had been dealing with epilepsy for most of my life, but it had been fairly controlled with my medication, giving me hope that I would be able to live a normal life. However during my senior year, everything changed. It started with the immense mental stress from my basketball coach. What was supposed to be my final season playing the game that had become a part of me, turned into overwhelming toxicity. I had already made up my mind before the season started that I wanted to transfer schools. A hand full of schools were willing to take me in, offering the support and opportunities I needed. All that stood in the way was my current coach releasing me. She refused to release me to the same conference, although they would be moving conferences the following year. This caused the tension between us to exasperate. At first, I thought I could handle it, pushing through as I always had, but it became more than I could bear.

The stress my coach put me under was relentless. The pressure of performing on the court wasn't my worry, her manipulative ways were a constant heavy mental strain that affected every part of me. She would only single me out for specific things, and my assistant coaches had brought that to her attention many times. The constant stress finally started to take a toll on my body. I was feeling sick constantly, and the more I tried to push through it, the worse it got. My epilepsy began to worsen again. I hadn't needed to see a neurologist consistently for some time, but it was clear that something chemically had changed. I could no longer ignore the seizures and symptoms that were becoming more frequent and severe.

I went back home to see a new neurologist, and that's when I was referred to the Cleveland Clinic Neurology. They are ranked nationally for adult epilepsy and neurology, and I have had the most amazing team of physicians since becoming a patient. It was there that I was diagnosed with a rare brain deformity called Polymicrogyria, that my pediatric neurologist had not caught. When I heard the diagnosis, it was essentially a relief to finally have answers after many years of what has been causing my seizures. The weight of my illness was overwhelming, and it was a stark reminder that epilepsy was something I would simply not "grow out of" like I had been told by previous neurologist as a child.

Learning that I had this rare condition did give me some sense of relief, I have always had this disorder but never knew what caused it until then. Having to go back to taking medicine added to my stress, but I knew I needed it. My body was shutting down on me, and my mind was overwhelmed with constant anxiety and depression. I had always been resilient, able to power through tough times but this time was different it felt like a jail sentence. No amount of grit or determination could fix what was happening inside me, I truly needed help.

Getting through that final basketball season was one of the hardest things I've ever had to do. My coach had stripped the happiness I had playing the sport I loved, making it harder each day to want to pick up a ball. Basketball was always my sanctuary and outlet, but I no longer felt that way being at Valpo. Every day felt like a battle just to keep going, both physically and mentally. The negativity from my coach didn't let up, and I couldn't escape the feeling that my body was betraying me. Yet, somehow with the support of some great friends I had met and the few teammates I was close with, I managed to push through. They helped me in ways they probably didn't even realize. Having the teammates that I was close with to vent to as they were going through similar experiences was relieving.

Nonetheless even with the support of friends, I knew that I couldn't handle everything on my own. My neurologist was doing everything possible to get my epilepsy back under control. He put me on several medications to help manage the seizures, but those medications came with their own set of challenges. The side effects were harsh, making even normal day-to-day tasks feel like colossal hurdles. I was often fatigued, emotionally drained, and felt like I was navigating through life in a haze. The medications were supposed to help me, but in many ways, I felt as if they weren't doing anything at all. Still, I knew they were necessary if I wanted any chance of regaining control over my brain.

As difficult as it was, seeking help was the best decision I could have made. I had always been someone who tried to push through pain and bottle everything up, both physical and emotional without asking for help. However there comes a point where no amount of inner strength can replace the need for outside support. Therapy became an essential part of my recovery my senior year. I was more willing to participate when I was older, than I was when I was younger. Talking to a professional about the mental and emotional toll that my health was taking on me allowed me to release the built-up frustrations and pain I had been carrying for so long. Having the access to a therapist on campus was vital to me, I was able to speak about things happening in real time and gain the tools I needed to get through those stressors.

The mental health aspect of my recovery was just as important as the physical side. For years, I had internalized so much of my pain especially with losing my father, bottling it up and refusing to let anyone in. I had been afraid of appearing weak or vulnerable, especially as someone who was known for their strength on and off the court. Therapy had showed me that vulnerability wasn't weakness, it was a necessary part of healing. I learned to be kinder to myself, to recognize that I didn't have to carry the weight of the world on my shoulders.

Recovery wasn't instant. It wasn't a linear path either, it is still a current journey of mine. There were days when I felt like I was making progress, only to have setbacks that made me question whether I would ever truly feel "better." Through it all, I began to realize that recovery isn't about being perfect or free of challenges, that is life. Learning how to navigate those challenges with the tools and support you've been given is how you get through those challenges. My neurologist, friends, family, and my therapist all played crucial roles in helping me get back to a place where I could function again. Therapy helped me process the trauma of my diagnosis and the emotional weight I had been carrying since my father's death. The more I talked about it, the lighter that weight felt. If there's one thing I've learned through this journey, it's that the process is not going to "fix" you but give you the proper tools to get back aligned. Finding ways to live and thrive, even with the challenges that life throws at you is the end goal.

IMPACT OF HIGHER EDUCATION

E ducation did far more than just provide knowledge, it broadened my perspective on life, teaching me how to see the world and interact with people in a way that is both empathetic and insightful. Over the years, education became a transformative force, not only shaping my professional path but also deeply influencing my personal relationships and how I understand people. The more I learned, the more I realized that knowledge isn't just about facts or what is in a text book, but about human connections. Through education, I was able to build bridges with people from various walks of life, learning to appreciate their experiences, challenges, and aspirations.

One of the most profound lessons that education taught me was how to engage with people. I have always been a shy individual so interacting with individuals outside of who I already knew was difficult. Early on I was so focused on academic success achieving high grades, excelling on exams, and gaining vital knowledge from what I was learning. However as time passed, my focus started to shift. I began to realize that the most important lessons were not only found in textbooks. They were found in the interactions I had with my classmates, professors, teammates, and even the individuals I encountered in my daily life. Learning became less about mastering content and more about understanding people. This shift in perspective changed how I related to others whether in a professional setting or personal relationships, I found that empathy and curiosity opened doors that knowledge alone could not.

The influence of my minor in psychology was particularly significant. Navigating in the world of psychology was an opportunity to dive deep into the human mind and understand why we think, feel, and behave the way we do. This was especially meaningful for me, given my own personal struggles. Living with epilepsy, coping with the loss of my father, and dealing with depression created layers of complexity in my life that I didn't fully understand. Truthfully sometimes I still don't understand. Studying psychology provided me with the tools to analyze my experiences and emotions in a way that made sense. I began to learn that my mind was not something working against me, but as something that could be understood, nurtured, and even trained.

Psychology gave me a framework to understand not just myself, but the people around me. I began to see how our thoughts and behaviors are influenced by a combination of factors like genetics, environment, past experiences, and social conditioning. It became easier to offer grace to others when they made mistakes or struggled with personal challenges. I realized that we are all products of our circumstances, and sometimes people act out of pain or fear rather than malice or incompetence. Unfortunately I learned this through experience with losing my father, acting out of emotion instead of thought. This understanding helped me foster stronger relationships, both personally and professionally.

The insights I gained from psychology also extended to my role as a coach. I coached basketball for about six years starting with elementary girls and ending with high school girls. Coaching became a way to mentor young athletes, helping them navigate both the physical and mental challenges of the game, while also teaching them life lessons. Working with kids was a unique experience, as it required a different kind of patience and understanding. Kids often face a mix of emotions and frustrations, and it was my job not only to help them improve their game but also to build their confidence and toughness. Coaching allowed me to use what I learned in psychology and life to help them manage their emotions, set goals, and overcome setbacks. It became clear to me that success in sports, much like in life, was as much about mental strength as physical ability.

As I worked with young athletes, I saw firsthand how important it was to understand the mental and emotional aspects of their lives. Many of them struggled with issues like anxiety, fear of failure, or the pressure to meet expectations. Through my experiences, I was able to identify these challenges and help them find ways to cope. Whether it was teaching them how to stay calm under pressure or encouraging them to adopt a growth mindset. Basketball has always been a form of therapy, where the court was a safe space for not only myself but also kids to work through their struggles.

Education shaped me as a person in a multitude of ways. Earning two associate's degrees, a bachelor's degree, and a master's degree while managing epilepsy, depression, and the lingering trauma from my father's death was no small feat. Each degree represented a victory over the different obstacles that tried to hold me back. It wasn't always easy to stay focused or motivated, especially when seizures would increase or when depression made it hard for me to collect a though. Nonetheless every time I completed a course or walked across a stage to receive a diploma, I was reminded of my own resilience and determination.

As I moved through each academic program or course, I knew that learning was preparing me for a career and becoming the best version of myself. Education gave me the tools to navigate life's challenges with more confidence and clarity. It taught me how to think critically, solve problems, and communicate effectively all skills that have served me well in every aspect of my life so far. Through my studies, I discovered that my true passion lay not just in engineering or sports, but in helping others whether through mentoring, advocacy, or just listening.

Coaching young athletes allowed me to see the world through their eyes full of possibilities but also filled with challenges. Working with kids requires a unique blend of patience, empathy, and leadership. You have to meet them where they are, understand their issues, and help them build confidence in themselves. Something that may seem small to me as an adult, may be detrimental to them. For many of these young athletes, sports are more than just a game, they are a way to prove to themselves and others that they can be good at what they do. I was able to use my education, especially my knowledge of psychology, to help them not only improve their athletic abilities but also develop resilience, discipline, and self-esteem.

Coaching became an extension of my own journey. Just as I had found solace in basketball after my father's death, I wanted to give these kids the same opportunity to use sports as a way to cope with their challenges. Whether they were struggling with family issues, school, or personal insecurities, I tried to create an environment where they could channel their energy into something positive. The court became a place of healing, growth, and self-discovery not just for them, but for me.

Education and having a disability has given me the tools to not only navigate my own challenges but to understand and help others do the same. Whether through coaching, mentoring, or simply being there for someone in need, I have learned that the most valuable thing we can offer each other is understanding. In many ways, my educational journey continues to this day. Every experience, every person I meet, every challenge I face adds to my understanding of the world and my place in it. I have come to see learning as a lifelong journey, one that doesn't end when you leave the classroom or the court. Each new opportunity to learn whether through formal education, personal experiences, or interactions with others offers a chance to grow. As I continue on this journey, I am constantly reminded of the power of education can transform lives.

REDISCOVERING MY PURPOSE

I have learned to find purpose by using my past traumas as strengths and as lessons, shaping the way I navigate through life today. The adversities I have faced, the pain, and the hardships are no longer seen as obstacles but as opportunities to grow and evolve. They've given me resilience, perseverance, and a unique perspective that I carry with me in all aspects of life. I've come to understand that the experiences we endure are what wire our brains and shape who we are. Trauma can either break you or build you, and after allowing it to break me for so long I made the conscious choice to allow it build me up.

The process of turning trauma into strength wasn't an easy one. There were times when it felt like the weight of everything I'd been through losing my father, battling epilepsy, struggling with depression, not getting along with my coach was too much to bear. It was easy to fall into a victim mindset, to allow the pain to define me. After many years of allowing the mental pain to break me down, I refused to let my past dictate my future. I started to see every challenge as an opportunity for growth, a chance to learn more about myself and the world around me. It wasn't an overnight transformation, but with time, I began to look at my trauma through a different lens.

I realized that experience both the good and the bad is what molds a person. Each experience we go through shapes our perspective, influencing how we see ourselves and how we interact with the world. Traumatic experiences, while painful, can be the most powerful teachers if we allow them to be. They force us to confront parts of ourselves we may not be comfortable with, to dig deep and find strength we didn't know we had. Through this process, I've learned that trauma can sometimes be a roadblock, but it can also be the foundation upon which we build a new, stronger version of ourselves.

One of the key lessons I've taken from my experiences is that success is what you as an individual defines it to be. For so long, I had a narrow view of success one that was tied to external validation, accolades, and achievements. Growing up, I was taught to measure success by how well I performed in school, being at the top, or winning games. While those accomplishments were important and fulfilling at the time, they weren't the full picture of what success truly means in life. It took years of reflection and personal growth to understand that success isn't one-size-fits-all. Everyone's success looks different on a personal scale, we all have different paths. You have to find the sound of your instrument, and learn to love that.

For me, success is now defined by inner peace and personal fulfillment. Overcoming the challenges that life throws at me and emerging on the other side as a better, more self-aware individual. Using my past experiences, even the painful ones, to help others who may be going through something similar. Success isn't about being perfect or never facing adversity it's about how you respond to those barriers, how you pick yourself up after a fall, or how you use your experiences to shape a more purposeful life negative or positive. Everyone's journey is unique, and therefore, everyone's version of success will look different.

I used to think that sports were the only way I could define success. For a long time, my identity was tied to being an athlete being recognized for my performance on the court, for my leadership, and for the discipline I consistently showed in games and practices. As time went on, I began to realize that there was more to me than just sports. I had to learn how to find positives about myself outside of the athletics. This was a difficult transition because basketball had been my escape, my coping mechanism, and my source of validation for so many years. I knew that if I wanted to grow as a person, I had to explore other facets of who I was.

One of the most significant shifts in my mindset was recognizing that my worth wasn't tied to my ability to perform in sports or having commending grades. For years, I had placed so much pressure on myself to excel in sports and academics that I hadn't taken the time to appreciate the other qualities that made me unique. I had to learn to see myself as more than just an athlete. I started to focus on my intellectual capabilities, my creativity, and my ability to connect with others on a deeper level. I began to appreciate the value of empathy, resilience, and compassion qualities that had always been there but had taken a backseat to my athletic and academic achievements.

Finding purpose outside of athletics allowed me to see myself in a new light. I started to view my past experiences as sources of strength instead of limitations. The resilience I developed on the court translated into other areas of my life, whether it was in my education, career, or personal relationships. I realized that the discipline, work ethic, and perseverance I had honed as an athlete were transferable skills that could help me succeed in any field. This realization gave me a sense of empowerment that I hadn't felt before, it made me understand that I was capable of much more than I had ever imagined.

As I continued to grow and evolve, I began to see the positive aspects of myself more clearly. I started to recognize that my ability to empathize with others, to listen to their struggles and offer support, was just as valuable as any physical skill I possessed. I learned to appreciate my emotional intelligence, my critical thinking, and my ability to problem-solve in difficult situations. These were qualities that had been there all along, but I had overlooked them in favor of focusing on my athletic and academic achievements. Embracing these aspects of myself gave me a deeper sense of purpose and fulfillment.

Learning to view my past traumas as strengths has been a pivotal part of my continuing journey. Rather than seeing the challenges I've faced as setbacks, I now view them as stepping stones. Every hardship I've encountered has taught me something valuable about myself and about life. I've learned to be patient with myself, to give myself grace when things don't go as planned, and to trust in my ability to overcome whatever comes my way. This mindset shift has allowed me to approach life with a sense of confidence and optimism, knowing that no matter what challenges lie ahead, I have the tools and the resilience to face them head-on.

My journey has also taught me the importance of helping others find their own strength in the face of adversity.

Through my own experiences, I've come to realize that we all have the capacity to turn our pain into power, but sometimes we need a little guidance or encouragement to do so. Whether it's through mentoring, coaching, or simply sharing my story, I've made it a priority to help others see that their struggles don't define them. We all have the ability to rewrite our narratives, to take control of our lives, and to find purpose in the midst of hardship. Ultimately, the most important lesson I've learned is that purpose comes from within. It's not anything that can be handed to you or found in external achievements, it's something that you have to cultivate through self-reflection, growth, and resilience.

For me, finding purpose has been about using my past traumas as a source of strength, learning from my experiences, and helping others do the same. Embracing my journey, with all of its ups and downs, and recognizing that every step along the way has contributed to the person I am today. Success, for me, now is defined by how I feel about myself, where I want to be on a personal scale and how I use my experiences to make a positive impact on the individuals around me. I've learned that true success is about finding peace within yourself, no matter what life throws your way. Revolving your pain into power, your trauma into strength, and your experiences into wisdom. Everyone's version of success looks different, and that is okay. What matters most is that you define it for yourself and that you find fulfill-ment in your own personal journey.

RISING BEYOND THE STORM

NAVIGATING THE UNSEEN

L iving with epilepsy is a journey that'll unfortunately never end. Epilepsy is a condition that doesn't always announce itself loudly, but it always makes its presence known through fatigue, uncertainty, and the constant attentiveness it demands. Usually known as the "invisible disorder" because you can't always physically see what I am going through. Personally, managing epilepsy has been a lifelong process of adapting, accepting, and finding the strength to thrive despite it. As both an individual living with a neurological condition and being an engineer who relies heavily on mental clarity and critical thinking, I've faced many moments of frustration, but also incredible growth in many aspects. Each day brings new lessons on resilience and originality.

One of the central pillars of managing epilepsy is medication. Despite knowing it is necessity, I've had a complicated relationship with it. The regimen I follow includes multiple pills a day fourteen at times. That many pills a day takes a mental toll on any individual. There are days where I can't tolerate another dose, where I resent the fog or fatigue that follows soon after.

I've struggled with staying consistent, sometimes going off the medication altogether out of frustration or a desire to feel "normal" or less foggy. Nevertheless, there are times I've stepped away from the prescribed routine, and was reminded of the reality I live with. The consequences of skipping medication can be serious and sometimes dangerous.

This ongoing battle is physical, mental, and an emotional journey. Taking medicine every day is a reminder that I have a condition I didn't ask for and can't control entirely on my own. Over time, I've begun to shift my mindset. I now try to view some of my medications as a tool rather than a burden; a necessary part of my toolkit for living well. I've had honest conversations with my neurologist and epilepsy psychologist about my resistance, and they've helped me understand the importance of balancing my mental health with my physical well-being. We've adjusted my treatment plan according to my concerns, to reduce side effects and improve how I feel on a daily basis, which has helped me stick with some of the medications a bit more frequently.

Even with the adjustments and progress, challenges remain. Sleep is both a constant struggle and one of the most essential pieces of managing epilepsy. When I don't get enough sleep or rest, I am trapped feeling unwell, a step behind, or in an aura. I am often caught in a cycle, the less sleep I get the more I don't feel well, the more I don't feel well the less sleep I get. I have learned to navigate my days knowing there is an increased chance I will be exhausted, but with great gratitude.

The headaches can also be brutal. Some days, they creep in slowly, while other days they hit hard and fast. The pain from these headaches can at times cause me to be hospitalized, forcing me to pause when all I want to do is keep moving forward. Thankfully, they now come in waves rather than being constant, and I am truly grateful for that.

Navigating this battle requires a myriad of things. It requires a constant check-in with myself physically, emotionally, and physically. Giving myself permission to rest when I need to, even when the world makes me feel guilty for slowing down. Finding ways to connect with others, even when my first instinct is to isolate. Being honest about my limits while also celebrating the victories, no matter how small they may seem. Some days that victory may be making it through work despite how bad I may feel. Other days it looks like taking my medications without hesitation, reminding myself it is for survival.

I am still learning to give myself grace. I am still learning to hold space for both the pain and the progress. I am still learning that it is okay to not have everything figured out, because life with epilepsy is never direct. It's a cycle of setback and growth, exhaustion and renewal. Some days, the balance feels impossible. Other days, I surprise myself with how much I can push myself to the limit. Through it all I remind myself that this journey, as brutal and exhausting as it can be, is also proof of my strength.

FINDING BALANCE

Professionally, I continue to thrive, bringing both my technical expertise and personal strength to my work. Personally, I continue to grow, becoming more self-aware, more compassionate, and more open to help and support. My condition has forced me to slow down at times, but it has also deepened my appreciation for the moments when I feel clear, confident, and strong. As a mechanical engineer, my work demands high-level problem-solving, mental endurance, and attention to detail. Whether I'm designing a component, troubleshooting a system, or collaborating with a team, I need to be mentally sharp.

I work in a field that thrives on precision, creativity, and the ability to problem solve in real time. My day to day responsibilities often include designing products, building things in AutoCAD, conducting test protocols, or collaborating with a versatile team. These tasks demand intense focus and mental clarity, especially when safety or performance is on the line. There's very little margin for error in engineering, which means I have to bring my best self to the table every single day. That sometimes becomes difficult when epilepsy is part of the equation. I don't always have control over how I feel or how clearly I can think. Some days, the seizures don't come, but the brain fog does. Most nights, I can't sleep more than five hours, and the exhaustion carries into the next day.

I've had to learn to work with what I have, to adjust how I approach my tasks when my brain isn't cooperating, and to advocate for myself when I need a break. I've developed systems that help me track and organize my workload better, like writing most things down, double-checking calculations even when I feel confident, and scheduling my most mentally demanding work for times when I typically feel clearest. It's a constant dance between efficiency and limitation, but one that I've learned to lead rather than follow. Epilepsy at times can get in the way of that. Brain fog can settle in at the worst times like while I am speaking, in the middle of a meeting, or while working through drawings. I've had moments where I know the answer to a question but can't quite grasp it because my mind is moving a step slower than usual.

On top of my work as a mechanical engineer, I've also pursued front-end development in my spare time. That decision was bred partly from curiosity, passion, and partially from the understanding that having multiple skill sets can provide a level of security and freedom that a single path might not offer. It's satisfying to build something from scratch with code and watch it all come to life. Writing code, debugging, and designing user interfaces can feel like solving puzzles, which I find both challenging and rewarding. On the other hand, it demands mental clarity. Long hours staring at a screen can be mentally taxing, especially when I'm already drained from a seizure or side effects from medication.

I've had to be very intentional about how I balance this work with everything else. I spend the first part of my day in the field for my mechanical engineering work, and then transition into front-end development projects in the evening at home. On good days, I feel energized by the shift in focus and on bad days, I have to recognize when I'm pushing myself too far. I've learned to say no when necessary, to pace myself, and to avoid the temptation to compare my productivity to others who aren't facing the same health challenges. Lack of sleep another side effect of my condition only adds to the difficulty of delay. That level of sleep deprivation would be challenging for anyone, but for someone with epilepsy, it can trigger seizures, impair memory, and make thinking feel like moving through quicksand. I've learned to recognize when my mind is foggy and try not to be so hard on myself on those particular days. I've also become an expert at structuring my day in a way that works with my brain instead of against it. I tackle high-focus tasks during my most alert hours and take breaks when I feel myself slipping into fatigue or delay.

Still, even with these obstacles, I've experienced tremendous success in my career. I've worked on exciting engineering projects, solved difficult technical problems, and earned recognition for many contributions. Finding ways to keep moving forward, even when the road gets tough is what helps me in my day to day life. Many people don't know I have this disorder, I have gotten so good at masking the symptoms. I experience the depression that often comes with long-term chronic disorder, causing a shift in mood a lot of the time. I've had moments of anxiety, especially when I can feel an aura the warning sign that a seizure might be coming or a smaller seizure before a larger one. That kind of anticipation is mentally exhausting. Imagine living with a condition where your brain, the very center of who you are, can betray you at any moment.

One of the most transformative steps I've taken is working with an epilepsy psychologist. Having someone who understands the condition from both a clinical and human perspective has made a huge difference. Together, we've talked through the frustrations, fears, and the emotional weight of living with epilepsy. We've explored coping strategies that help me feel more grounded and less overwhelmed. I've also learned to set boundaries in my life and work, to not push myself beyond my limits just to prove I can and to not be afraid to speak up when I am not feeling well.

Over time, I've developed healthier ways to manage the mental toll. I've stopped bottling things up and started talking more openly about my condition or what may be bothering me. That alone has been one of the most freeing actions I've taken. Sharing my story has not only helped me process my own experience but has also allowed others to relate, support me, and learn from what I'm going through. There are times when I feel like some of the people closest to me do not care, and I was hurt for a long time. However, I learned that even if I touch just one person with my story that still makes a difference, regardless of who it is.

THE SOUND OF
COURAGE

Perhaps the most important change in my journey has been the shift from isolation to community. For a long time, I kept my epilepsy a secret. I didn't want people to treat me differently or see me as weak. People have a bad habit of making excuses for individuals with disorders, illnesses, or diseases and I never wanted anyone feeling sorry for me. Nonetheless, hiding it only made things harder for me. Eventually, I made the decision to join an epilepsy support group called Empowering Epilepsy and that changed a lot in my life.

Being part of a community of people who understand what you're going through is incredibly empowering. There's a certain type of comfort in knowing you're not alone, in hearing others describe the same struggles you thought were yours alone. We share stories, tips, frustrations, victories, and speak to neurologist from all over the United States. We cheer each other on and lift each other up. That community gave me the courage to accept my condition more fully and talk about it more openly in my daily life. Acceptance doesn't mean resignation. Acceptance means acknowledging the reality of my condition without letting it define me. I've stopped comparing myself to people who don't live with epilepsy, they will never understand and I get that now. I've embraced the fact that my brain works differently but also effectively and that is okay. There's strength in difference. There's wisdom in struggle and there's power in being vulnerable and authentic.

Today, I manage my epilepsy with a combination of medical care, mental health support, lifestyle adjustments, and acceptance. I'm not perfect, and some days are harder than others. However, I have built a foundation that allows me to keep moving forward. Learning to be more resilient has gotten me through some of my worst days. I'm proud of the person I've become through this journey. Although I make managing epilepsy look easy on the outside it isn't easy, but has taught me lessons I couldn't have learned any other way. Epilepsy has shown me the importance of balance, patience, and perspective. It's pushed me to develop inner strength, lean on others when needed, and always keep moving forward even if it's just one step at a time.

Each role I carry comes with its own expectations, responsibilities, and challenges. Juggling them all while managing a neurological condition means I've had to develop unique coping strategies and a mindset that allows me to not just function, but to excel. It hasn't always been easy, and there have been moments of exhaustion, discouragement, and self-doubt. Over time, I've found a rhythm that works for me a rhythm that includes grace, adaptation, and persistent determination.

Living with epilepsy adds a layer of complexity to everything I do. The seizures themselves are the easiest part, it is the level of unpredictability, the emotional toll, and the effort it takes to function normally when my brain feels anything but normal. I've gone through periods where I tried to pretend it wasn't affecting me, where I pushed myself to keep up appearances. The truth is, that approach always ends up costing me more in the long run physically, mentally, and emotionally. What I've come to realize is that balance is about knowing when to shift gears, when to rest, and when to push forward. I've had to learn how to prioritize, how to manage my energy more than my time, and how to build a support system that allows me to thrive.

Some of the most important changes I've made are internal. I've stopped feeling guilty for needing rest or not feeling well. I've stopped punishing myself for being slower on certain days, something I can't help. I've accepted that I can't control everything, and that doing my best will look different depending on the day. That mindset shift has allowed me to be more present in everything I do. Whether I'm working on a mechanical drawing, coding a new website, or managing my health, I try to bring the same level of intention and integrity. I may have limitations, but I also have many valuable strengths. My focus, discipline, flexibility have all sharpened precisely because of those limitations. They've taught me how to approach problems from different angles, how to stay calm under pressure, and how to stay committed to growth even when progress is slow.

Another key to maintaining balance has been the relationships I've built along the way. I don't do this alone. I've had

mentors, teammates, friends, family, and healthcare providers who've supported me, challenged me, and helped me stay
grounded. I've been honest with people I trust about my condition and what I need in order to succeed. That transparency has
allowed me to build deeper connections and to feel less isolated,
especially with my mom. There were times when I was younger
when I felt like she just wasn't hearing how I felt because of her
worry, rightfully so. I started to advocate for myself and open my
mouth about how I felt, and she learned to listen.

Being a part of an epilepsy community has also given me
strength. Knowing that others are going through similar battles has helped me stay encouraged, and it's reminded me that
strength is about continuing despite the struggle. There are
moments where I feel completely in sync when I finish a successful project, solve a complex coding issue, or make it through
a week with no major health setbacks. In those moments, I feel
unstoppable. Even in the harder moments when I'm drained,
foggy, or discouraged, I've learned to trust that the cycle will shift
again, that clarity will return, and that progress is still possible.
I've also found ways to incorporate more rest into my routine.
Not just sleep, which is already hard to come by, but intentional
rest taking, maintaining a workout schedule, meditating, or
spending time in spaces that bring me peace. These practices
may seem small, but they've helped me recharge and maintain
the stamina needed to sustain all these roles.

The truth is, I don't have a perfect formula for balance, it
is about what works for you as an individual. What I have is a
deep commitment to making it work, to doing the best I can

with the tools I have, and to constantly learning what balance means for me. It's an evolving process, one that shifts with every new project, every seizure, and every personal breakthrough. Some weeks are heavier on engineering, others on recovery. Some days I'm immersed in lines of code, other days I'm focused on my health or connecting with others in the epilepsy community. The balance isn't always equal, but it is always intentional. That intention is what allows me to live fully in every role I play.

There's a certain power in knowing that you're carrying something difficult and still moving forward. That power has been my anchor. It's what fuels my passion for engineering, for technology, and for helping others. It's what keeps me grounded when I feel like everything is too much. I may be living with epilepsy, but I'm also living with purpose. I'm a builder, a thinker, a problem solver. I'm someone who's found a way to integrate the highs and lows of my condition into a meaningful and productive life. That, to me, is the true definition of balance and success.

Living with epilepsy has changed the way I view the world, my purpose, and the impact I want to make. For years, I stayed silent about my condition, hiding it from nearly everyone around me. It was something I didn't feel comfortable sharing not out of shame necessarily, but out of fear. People can be extremely cruel and I wanted to avoid those type of interactions. I didn't want to be treated differently, pitied, or underestimated. I didn't want epilepsy to be the first thing people saw when they seen me. So I coped quietly, managing seizures behind closed doors, battling fatigue in silence, and navigating the mental and emotional toll as privately as possible.

With time, experience, and growth, I've come to understand that my silence wasn't protecting me it was limiting me. It was keeping me from connecting with others who needed to hear my story and keeping me from accepting myself fully. Now, I see epilepsy not just as a personal challenge but as a platform a way to educate, inspire, and advocate for others who live with the same condition.

Over the past few years, I've tried speaking more openly about my condition. I have shared not just the facts, but the lived experiences the restless nights, the brain fog, the frustration of taking multiple medications every single day, the struggle to stay focused in a demanding profession when my body and mind are not always cooperating. These moments, while they may seem simple on the surface, represent the quiet strength that people living with epilepsy develop over time. By putting my story out there, I've started to connect with others who walk similar paths. People from different backgrounds and professions have messaged me saying they never thought someone like them could speak up about it. It's helped me realize how much need there is for representation and openness in the epilepsy community.

Talking about my experiences publicly has also helped me heal in ways I didn't expect. Every time I open up, I feel a little more free. Every conversation, every post, every message exchanged with someone who says, "Thank you for sharing that, it's exactly how I feel," chips away at the isolation I once carried so heavily. It's powerful to know that by being honest about my pain, I might be giving someone else permission to be honest about theirs. That kind of connection is the beginning of change. It's what advocacy is really about raising awareness, but also building community and letting people know they're not alone. Beyond that, it's about owning your own narrative, rather than letting it be defined by silence, stigma, or misunderstanding.

The more I opened up, the more I saw how few platforms exist where people living with epilepsy are leading the conversation. Medical professionals and researchers talk about us all the time, but rarely with us. There's a gap in the way our stories are told, and I feel a responsibility to help fill that gap. So I began writing this book that documents not only my journey but the greater experience of living with epilepsy in a world that often fails to see invisible conditions. My goal with this book is simple, to reach people who feel unseen or unheard living with epilepsy. To give them a voice, even if they haven't found the courage to speak yet. To offer validation, support, and an honest reminder that their life still has value and meaning. Even living with epilepsy we have the power to do many things, and I want to make others aware of that.

At the same time, I've been working on developing an epilepsy resource website. I envisioned a platform where information meets lived experience. While there are plenty of websites with general facts about epilepsy, very few provide a true sense of community or center the voices of people who live with it daily. I want my website to be a hub for those living with epilepsy, those newly diagnosed, caregivers, and allies. It will include articles on managing symptoms, coping strategies, mental health support, medication tips, sleep hygiene, recipes, and lifestyle advice written by and for people who live this reality. I also want to highlight underrepresented voices people of color, young professionals, athletes, students whose journeys with epilepsy are often left out of mainstream narratives. Through interviews, blog posts, and community forums, I want this website to be more than just a collection of resources, it should feel like a digital support group, a safe place to learn, vent, connect, and grow.

Even more than that, I want this advocacy work to extend into the physical world. I've started exploring opportunities to speak at conferences, schools, epilepsy awareness events, and corporate workshops. I believe the most powerful form of education is storytelling when people hear a real human voice attached to a condition, it becomes harder to ignore or reduce to a stereotype. I want to speak to young people and let them know that epilepsy doesn't mean the end of your dreams. I want to speak to professionals in high-stress fields like engineering and tech to show that it's possible to succeed even with medical challenges. I want to speak to caregivers and medical providers to help them see beyond symptoms and into the lives of the people they care for. These are not just elevated goals they're actionable steps I've begun taking to expand my impact and transform advocacy from something I write about into something I live.

The idea of speaking publicly used to terrify me. Not because I don't know what to say, but because I feared being seen as weak, different, or incapable. I now realize that being open about my condition is one of the strongest things I can do for myself and for others. Every time I speak up, I hope to make it easier for someone else to do the same. If I can stand in front of a room of people and talk about what it means to live with epilepsy without apologizing, minimizing, or hiding then maybe the next person who's struggling will find the courage to stand up as well.

I also hope my journey shows that you can be more than your diagnosis. Yes, I live with epilepsy. but I am also an engineer, a creative thinker, a mentor, a problem solver, an athlete, and a fighter. I've succeeded in my career thus far, excelled in academics, and contributed to my community all while dealing with something that could have easily sidelined me. That's the message I want to amplify not that epilepsy defines us, but that we can define what our lives look like in spite of it. Advocacy is showing the strength, joy, determination, and the full humanity of people living with chronic conditions. I want to rewrite the narrative and show the world that people with epilepsy are not fragile, broken, or helpless we are resilient, resourceful, and powerful.

There's still a long way to go. Stigma still exists, access to care is unequal, and too many people are suffering in silence. Change doesn't happen all at once. It starts with a post, a conversation, a shared story, a website, a book, a classroom visit. Each step creates a domino effect. That is what keeps me going. Even on the hard days, even when I feel drained from lack of sleep or frustrated by brain fog or discouraged by side effects, I remind myself that what I'm doing matters. That my story matters. That the work I'm doing on a daily basis can and will help others navigate this complex journey with more hope and less fear.

I never thought epilepsy would be the thing that pushed me to speak up. Sometimes the hardest things in life end up shaping you in the most unexpected ways. They reveal your strength, clarify your purpose, and connect you with people who make the journey worth it. That's what epilepsy has done for me. If I can use my voice, my platform, and my experience to lift someone else up to help them feel seen, heard, and empowered then every seizure, every hard night and every moment of doubt will have led to something meaningful.